What's Food Got To Do With It?

A Love Letter to Americans about Self-Love and Nutrition

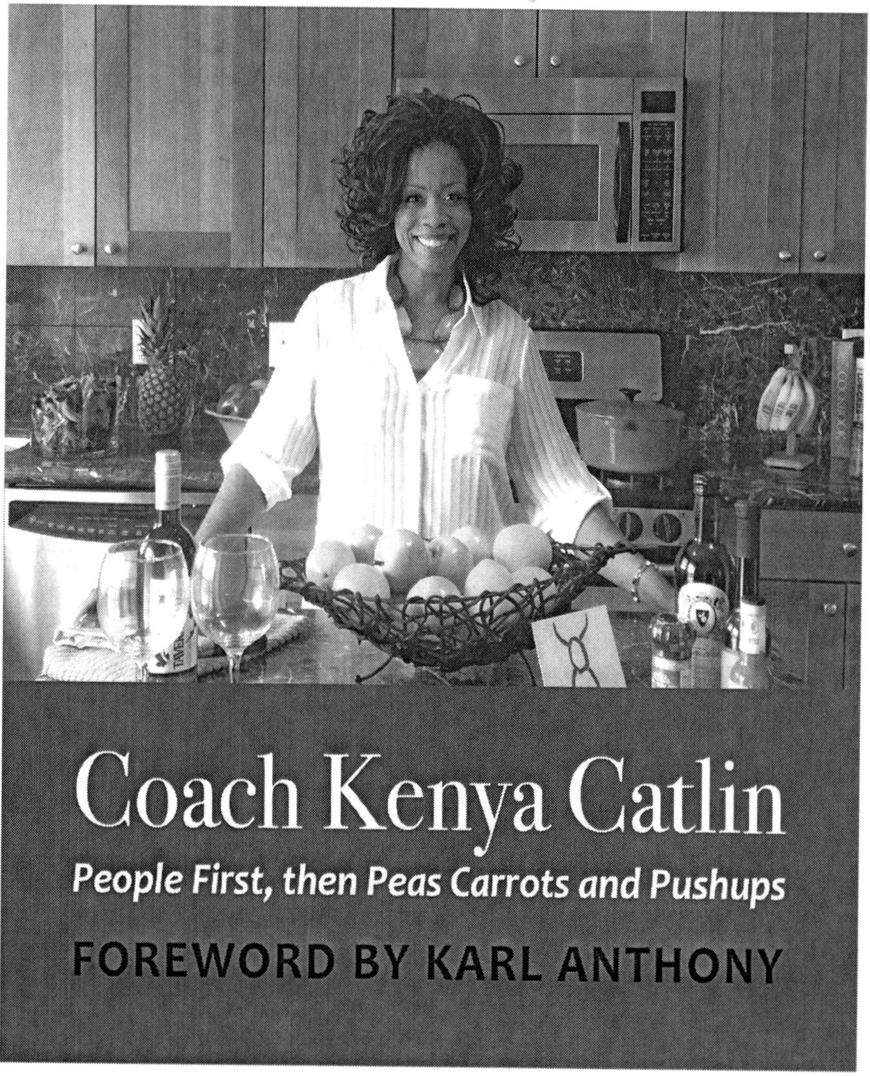

Coach Kenya Catlin

People First, then Peas Carrots and Pushups

FOREWORD BY KARL ANTHONY

What's Food Got To Do With It?

A Love Letter to Americans about Self-Love and Nutrition

Volume I 2015

By Coach KENYA Catlin
People First, then Peas Carrots and Pushups

Copyright©2015 by Coach KENYA

All rights reserved. No part of this book may be reproduced in any form or by any electronic or mechanical means, including information storage and retrieval systems, without permission in writing from the author. For information, contact KenyaCatlin@gmail.com

The content of this book is for general instruction only. Each person's physical, emotional, and spiritual condition is unique. The instruction in this book is not intended to replace or interrupt the reader's relationship with a physician or other professional. Please consult your doctor for matters pertaining to your specific health and diet.

All rights reserved. No part of this publication may be reproduced, distributed, or transmitted in any form or by any means, including photocopying, recording, or other electronic or mechanical methods, with prior written permission of the publisher or author, except in the case of brief quotations embodied in critical reviews and certain other noncommercial uses permitted by copyright law. For permission requests, email the publisher or author at KenyaCatlin@gmail.com or send your request to info@mybodydivine.com

To contact the author, visit
WWW.MYBODYDIVINE.COM

ISBN 9780692481257

Printed in the United States of America

DEDICATION

This book is dedicated to all God's children, as a reminder that we are all connected and the better we understand this truth the better the world will be.

Expressly
Willie Jones (Grand paw)
You are still the wind beneath our wings.

Cylanthia Lee (Mama)
Behind all the craziness there are many layers of love.

Karl Anthony Catlin aka Focus
My # 1 son whose leadership and care has taught me.

Kristopher A.S. Catlin aka Freedom
Mama's baby and one of the most loving people on the planet; keep loving there is room.

Lilah Marie Atkinson-Catlin and Julius Paul Catlin
My G-Babies
You have given me a whole new capacity for love.

CONTENTS

Acknowledgements 5

How to Use This Book.. 7

Introduction.. 8

Chapter 1: The Greatest Love of All Self-Love............................11

Chapter 2: The Connection between Food and Chronic Illness....... 23

Chapter 3: Preventing Chronic Illness...47

Chapter 4: Food as Medicine..53

Chapter 5: Nutrition Anyone?..67

Chapter 6: Financial Fitness...77

Chapter 7: Exercise is a Bonus..83

Chapter 8: Exactly What to Do Now! 89

Quotes & Notes..99

References...100

About the Author..101

ACKNOWLEDGEMENTS

It has been a long journey to here. Looking back, I could have arrived at this point long ago but I never would have experienced the people, places and things I did along the way. So I am grateful.

I would especially like to thank:

My BODY DIVINE™ clients for allowing me to grow and learn from you; your faith and support anchored me.

The staff, fellow coaches and volunteer's time is the most precious gift thanks for sharing yours with me.

The people of the Cities of Chicago and San Antonio the differences in the two cities confirm how we are so much alike.

Every friend & foe that has crossed my path; you have helped to shape who I am. And I love that.

Anyone who has ever supported my products and services.

Wellness warriors all around the globe.

FOREWORD

It amazes me that so many people are not educated about the importance of nutrition in maintaining a healthy lifestyle. The aches, pains, energy levels and even thoughts are often a direct connection to the nutrition that we use to fuel our bodies, mind and spirit. This concept is so rudimentary that people often overlook it. For some a healthy lifestyle can seem esoteric like a privilege that only a select few can attain. That perception is indeed false. Taking steps to better your health is not only simple, but necessary if you intend on living a vibrant and productive life. As a young aspiring entertainer, I have to maintain the ability to not be shaken by the twist and turns of life. I don't always know what lies ahead but I realize I have a much better chance of facing challenges with a healthy body, mind and spirit. The foods you chose ultimately add life to your years and years to your life. This is precious time that can be spent with family, friends, and doing what you love. Today we are witnessing a large number of people egress due to poor lifestyle choices. The fuel we use has enormous influence on what we do and what we fail to do.

– Karl Anthony
Writer/Entertainer

HOW TO USE THIS BOOK

Set an Intention

Get clear on how you got where you are. If you are doing great, keep doing more of the same. If you have challenges, think about the areas you wish to develop and slowly take steps in the direction of change. Know that time and consistency is the key to making your intentions become a reality and on your way to greatness pick someone else up for the ride.

Have Fun

In this book, you will find concepts in self-love and proper nutrition. Choose the concepts that you can envision yourself doing. Remember all the concepts are connected. Then take a honest look at the community that you are responsible to serve and ask yourself, can I play a part in making it better. Trust that when you are doing good-good will come.

Be Open to Change

A habit can make or break you. Do not try and get rid of all your bad habits. Slowly begin replacing them with good habits. And do not beat yourself up if you fall off. When you fall, fall forward. In time the good will outweigh the bad. That is called balance.

Do a Little at a Time

In this book, you will be re-introduced to concepts you know to be true. Recommit to not just knowing concepts but the practice of doing. Everyday strive to glorify God, help others and do what makes you happier and healthier.

INTRODUCTION

Fast forward to my return to Chicago, it is abundantly clear self-love and proper nutrition must be taught. Americans must take their health more serious and learn the connection between what we eat, think, and do and how it affects our health, our neighborhoods, our finances and our connection to all of life.

Far too many people suffer and die prematurely from preventable diseases. We cannot face the problems that plague our communities if we are not well in our mind, body, and finances.

The solution is a simple proposition; practice self-care and proper nutrition at a basic level and results will follow.

My intention in this book is to encourage everyday people who manage tight schedules and limited budgets to incorporate these practices into their lives as a means of leading a happier, healthier and disease free life.

In this book, I will identify problems by raising awareness but more potently we will look at practical solutions to grant anyone who wishes more health, happiness and wholeness in their life.

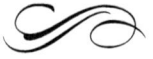

*If your God
is mighty enough to ignite the sun,
could it be that he is mighty enough
to light your path?*[1]

—Max Lucado

CHAPTER 1

SELF-LOVE

What comes first the chicken or the egg? Although there are very compelling theories for both arguments on which came first, no person really knows the answer. In relationship to self-love and proper nutrition; which comes first? Do you love yourself enough to properly nurture your body or do you nurture your body to gain more self-love?

Frankly, I am not sure it matters. What does matter is either way provides a great start; so pick one!

According to Gallup surveys taken over the past 15 years, 33 percent of Americans over the age of eighteen are born again Christians. Numerically this translates into 59 million Christians or one out of three adults who experienced a turning point. On the surface this sounds good but in actuality this is a tragedy because the greatest revival in history has taken place yet yielded no positive change in how we as a society live.

In some cases, Americans are more segregated than ever before. The gap between the rich and poor is wider than ever. Our focus on children and the elderly is not a priority, crime has become fashionable and sex without commitment is as American as apple pie.

How is it possible to have access to such a true and loving God yet be so deficient in areas that create happiness and wholeness? How is it possible to have a revolution without a change?

The answers lie in SELF-LOVE.

By definition self-love is having regard for one's own well-being; a happiness void of vanity, conceit or narcissism. In this book, I use the word self-care please note that self-love and self-care are interchangeable by definition.

In my private Health Coaching practice in Chicago with weight loss clients it has been especially challenging for some clients to follow basic recommendations. Simple instructions like eat more vegetables, consume three meals per day or just showing up for scheduled workouts seem like an insurmountable task. Though lovely people these clients had so many deterrents in their lives. Many of them skipped breakfast, worked long hours without food or water, made atrocious food choices when they did eat, got very little sleep and repeated these behaviors over again the next day for a job that they complained about. If you examine this behavior closely it almost sounds like behaviors you would expect from people who live in third world countries... Not America!

These behaviors may not seem like a big deal until I tell you each person who exhibited these behaviors was overweight or obese, suffered from at least two chronic illnesses and managed a minimum of two toxic relationships in their lives usually one at work and one at home. Mostly importantly, each person had very little or no support when it came to living a healthy lifestyle. As a result most did very little to give back to the community they lived in (with the exception of going to work and or church) and most did not have a positive outlook on much of anything. In essence, people are simply going through the motions and these are the good people.

My work in Chicago has proven to be the hardest and the most rewarding.

SELF-LOVE SOLUTIONS

They were just doing what they never learned. The idea of a hot bath, a good book and a great meal competed with learned behaviors like morning coffee with eight sugars on an empty stomach and an evening with fried chicken and a bottle of wine. My work was cut out for me; I quickly shifted my focus to raising awareness of how to love and nourish ourselves. From there we can tackle weight loss, chronic illnesses and the many other factors that shape who we are and who we will become.

For many years I worked for American Airlines where safety is a number one priority. At every departure the flight attendants would give the required safety briefing. In the event of an emergency your oxygen mask will deploy. If you are seated next to a small child or elderly person please secure your oxygen mask first and then offer assistance to your neighbor. It is not rocket science to help yourself so that you can help others.

Men nurture your bodies, mind and spirit so that you can direct your families. Women nurture your bodies, mind and spirit so that you may support your families. Children nurture your bodies, mind and spirit; so you have the power to be the first generation to help your elders and children to lead healthy lives.

LEARNING TO LOVE YOURSELF

I believe the children are the future. Teach them well and let them lead the way. Show them all the beauty they possess inside. Give them a sense of pride to make it easier...

The greatest love of all is to learn to love yourself. Imagine how much different the world would be if each person possessed a burning love for themselves. Loving others would be so much simpler. Loving yourself takes place in the womb. Unborn children can feel the effects of their environment. Thoughts, feelings and personalities begin to form in the womb. Once a child is born, parents and grandparents play a role in developing a child's sense of self. The child then begins to experience the normal growing pains of life such as transitioning into school, making friends, deciding what to be when they grow up and dealing with the milestones of pre-adolescence and adolescence. These years shape a person's life forever.

Nowadays support from parents, grandparents and the community are fading in some areas and nonexistent in others. Children are not being conceived out of love. Having two loving parents in the home has become the exception and not the rule. According to polls almost half of American children are raised in nontraditional households. In fact, grandparents have taken on the role of parenting in the absence of the biological parents. Make no mistake people are doing the best they can. The truth is the karmic cycles of family and community are broken. So with all that is out of whack, how do you learn to love yourself?

Love is a decision you make every day. It sounds simple and it really is. Every morning you get up and you make a decision to make your bed or not. It does not matter whether you own the most beautiful sheets or whether your sheets are tattered and torn; you can care for them and treat them as if they have value. Loving yourself and others works the same way. You have to make a decision.

It is foolish to think that everyone will jump out of bed daily with a loving spirit especially in the midst of soaring unemployment rates, high crime, broken relationships, lack of energy from poor nutrition, chronic illnesses on the rise and a host of other problems.

In order to thrive (not just hang on) you are going to need to recruit some help in these areas.

HAPPINESS

The laws of quantum psychics suggest that two opposing objects cannot occupy the same space at the same time; this is true of fear and faith or in this case happiness and sadness. It is impossible to be happy when you are sad or sad when you are happy. If you do not believe me watch a funny movie that makes you laugh, listen to your favorite song or even have someone tickle you. It would be impossible to feel down and up at the same time. Make a conscious decision daily to make up your bed with happiness.

THINK POSITIVE

Another habit of people practicing self-love is positive thinking even when it is gloomy. Positive people provide light to those around them and when they cannot be the light they find their way to the light.

It has amazed me how many conversations I have encountered in coffee shops, grocery stores and in my overall travels that are problem based. Do not be that person who brings gloom and doom into the room. Be the light and if your light is not shining bright at the moment it is okay to get a re-charge from someone whose light is bright. We are products of our environment and the people we spend the balance of our time with. It is very easy to get caught up in the gloom and doom syndrome of life. Ask yourself if the words you offer are encouraging and solution based. If your words are encouraging, that's great. If your words are not, it is ok to be silent and just observe those around you. In doing so, you will raise your awareness of the energy around you and become better at speaking solutions rather than problems.

In no way am I naive I am very clear about the conversations taking place in our communities. Children are misbehaving, the boss is irritating, co-workers are back-stabbing, and the lines are too long at the grocery counter. I am not suggesting that being positive will be easy all the time and I certainly do not mean to down play what you experience on a daily basis but the first step starts with raising your awareness and making a concentrated effort to be the light in every circumstance. If every person would practice this one concept alone our communities would change in an instant.

GRATITUDE

God has not promised me sunshine. That is not the way it is going to be. But a little rain mixed with God's sunshine and a little pain makes me appreciate the good times...

As a teenager, I had a plethora of friends from a variety of backgrounds. Somehow I tended to stray towards the bad boys and bad girls. They just seemed like more of a fit and more fun, which makes this next story so precious. A friend invited me to church one Sunday and I accepted her invitation. Now let's be clear, during my entire young adult wheeling and dealing, I have always been plugged in and had a great reverence for God. Sunday mornings have always been special to me. I have always had a strong sense of my spirituality. As the story goes, it was a small church and I remember the people being a bit more holy than I was accustomed to but, never the less, my friend was excited about Jesus and so was I. I remember the choir singing Lionel Richie's song – Father's Help your Children (Jesus is Love) the other song selection was Be Grateful by Walter Hawkins & Family. I still remember that day and those songs as though it were yesterday.

Be grateful for what you have the tangible and intangible. Once you truly get this concept your world will open. The smallest and biggest things in life you will appreciate.

SELF-ESTEEM

In undergraduate school my major was marketing. I recall we spoke in length about the product life cycle. In simple terms the product life cycle suggest that when you introduce a product to market it goes through four stages; introduction, growth, maturity and decline. Once a product reaches maturity the next step is decline. Most companies find ways to reinvent their product or service in an effort to prevent decline. Communities must reinvent themselves and their marketing agenda. Your community marketing plan determines in many ways how you see yourself. As an individual you may possess great esteem but if your community esteem is lacking it makes it hard for you to stay on your square. The notion that we really are connected is a real one. The most effective way to build self-esteem is too start with yourself then others especially those around you. The connection between the two creates an energy that is bad, indifferent or good. I don't have to suggest that "Good Energy" is the square that you want to be on. You will also want everyone in your circle to have good energy it will only make your life more manageable.

In my Health Coaching practice, I have a company philosophy - do the parts you like and are passionate about... the rest will come. Use this passion to spread love, peace, honor to God, family, community and the world. This is done by pushing solutions, not problems. Think of ways (energy) to make things better not worse and remember that words are powerful ways of thinking out loud. The bible says, we have the power of life and death in the tongue. Grandma says, "If you ain't got nothing good to say then don't say nothing at all."

These new aged philosophies compliment not only what you say to others but primarily what you say to yourself. What you say to yourself will be the building blocks of the energy you extend to others.

LEARNING TO LOVE OTHERS

The Bible says, in Hebrews 13:2 do not forget to show hospitality to strangers, for by so doing some people have shown hospitality to angels without knowing it. This is big. It is a good practice to look at strangers and treat them as if they were angels. The truth is if we would treat strangers with value we would harvest so much more value for our family, friends and neighbors. Treating every person you encounter as a piece of your life's puzzle. Knowing that there are eight billion people on the planet maybe just maybe a half dozen or so are here to help you navigate through this maze we call life. Not all are meant to stay for the entire journey and that is okay but we must make the initial connection to treat our encounter with people with value for without it we have very little chance at succeeding and growing.

EYE CONTACT AND A SMILE

The first step in treating strangers as if they are angels is connecting through basic salutations like saying hello or smiling. In my adult years I have noticed a lack of hospitality when it comes to simply greeting one another. In fact it amazes me that people who frequent the same places rarely make connections with people they see several times each week. People genuinely have no idea what a person they see does for a living. Even people who attend the same church and sit next to one another have never exchanged names. There is really no way to justify this disconnect. We must do better as a society. Over the years, I have adopted themes or mantras to live by. For instance one year a friend and I discussed giving people value. What if each of us would value other people around us? Value your carpenter as a great carpenter. Tell others about his great work and speak light into any conversations about his work. Talk up his work and refer him to others knowing that your words carry great influence. Now let's be clear; if we are going to follow this mantra, let's make sure truth is a part of the equation. If he is a lousy carpenter suggest to him to take a class to become better at his craft. Be sure to express this truth to him in a loving way privately. The point is, we need to uplift others with our smallest actions and words. This is a great way to practice loving others and giving them value at the same time.

STRIKING UP A CONVERSATION

A great way to create a connection with strangers you see around you every day is by striking up a conversation. It starts with a single hello then who knows where a conversation can take you from there. Some of my greatest connections have been made through talking with a stranger. Be careful not to have conversations out of gloom and doom syndrome. It is very easy to get into superficial conversations and to talk about all that is negative in the world. In striking up conversations I have noted some of the things people say to cut their own throats, not realizing that our thoughts turn into words and our words become our reality. Here are a few examples of negative things people have become accustom to saying and what they can be replaced with:

What We Are Saying	What We Should Be Saying
I'm tired	I'm working on getting more rest
I'm broke	I'm working on abundance
He/she is bad	Children are gifts
It is what it is	It is what I make it
I'm hanging in there	I'm soaring like an eagle
I don't have any women friends	I embrace sharing with women
Nobody cares about the hood	It's up to me to care for my neighborhood
I ain't going to settle down with one man/woman	In my heart I desire a committed relationship

If you are stuck speaking negative words you undoubtedly need a new marketing plan. You and you alone are responsible for changing your view of how you see yourself and how others see you through what you say.

Do not become that person complaining in the summer that it is too hot and in the winter that it is too cold. Find ways to extract what is good and produce solutions out of every situation. This is how individuals and communities grow.

EVERYBODY HAS CHALLENGES

Every community faces challenges at some point. What gets people past their challenges is their ability to speak and then act on solutions. It helps tremendously when everyone can come together in solidarity to push out favorable outcomes.

No man is an island...[2]

- John Donne

CHAPTER 2

The Connection

As I write this section I am experiencing an overwhelming sense of commitment to get this right. I do not want to mess this up. As I read through the literature from the World Health Organization (WHO), Green Facts, Centers for Disease Control (CDC), and National Center for Biotechnology Information and rely on my personal experience as a Health Coach, it is my knowing that people must be taught self-care and proper nutrition.

FOOD AND CHRONIC ILLNESS

We are all so connected in word and deed. This concept you will hear me repeat over and over again. If you could grasp this simple concept you could change your life and the lives of those around you. Another concept that must be addressed is the connection between illness and what we put in our bodies. As a practicing Health Coach it never ceases to amaze me that some people just get it and others fall way short of the goal. I do not judge, in fact quite the contrary. One important premise for this book is to spread the word about our relationship with food knowing we can do better. We can eat better.

I will explore a few theories as to why the margins are so huge in certain communities. Most importantly we will look at how to close those margins so that everyone who chooses has an opportunity to prevent illness and seek wellness in every area of their lives. After all isn't good health what you want?

WHAT IS CHRONIC ILLNESS?

By definition chronic illness is a long lasting condition that can be controlled but not cured. Chronic illness affects the population worldwide. As described by the CDC, chronic illness is the leading cause of death and disability in the United States. A few common examples of chronic illnesses are arthritis, asthma, breast cancer, multiple sclerosis, diabetes, epilepsy, glaucoma, heart disease, obesity and overweight.

COACH KENYA'S DEFINITION OF CHRONIC ILLNESS

The medical definition of chronic illness is a great one. However I would like to break down the definition into everyday terms that anyone can understand. First know that chronic illness does not always kill you first and for a large majority of people it can linger for years and wreak havoc in your body, mind, spirit, finances, family and just about everything you do or cannot do due to chronic illness controlling every aspect of your existence. By all means look at chronic illness as a disability with the ability to debilitate even the mightiest of spirits. The second point I would like to emphasize is chronic illness is preventable and manageable. In my health coaching practice, I encounter many people that get diagnosed and play right into the hands of that diagnoses. Hear this loud and clear: YOU ARE NOT YOUR DIAGNOSES! Say these words to yourself – "My body is strong and has incredible healing power – it is up to me to manifest the power from within using every primary and secondary food at my disposal."

LET'S LOOK AT THE FOOD FACTS

Green Facts, an online publication, released a summary on the effects of diet and nutrition in the prevention of chronic disease. In context the finding concluded that as a result of the way we eat and live some chronic diseases are increasingly affecting both developed and developing countries. Diet related chronic diseases – such as obesity, diabetes, cardio vascular disease, cancer, dental disease and osteoporosis are the most common causes of death in the world and present a great burden for society.

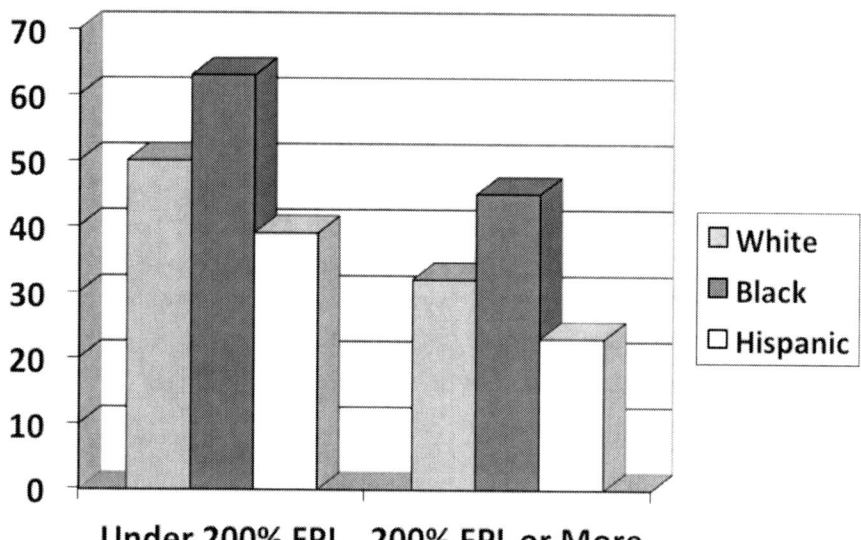

Chart 1. Percentage of adults ages 18 to 64 with any chronic condition or disability. The Commonwealth Fund.[3]

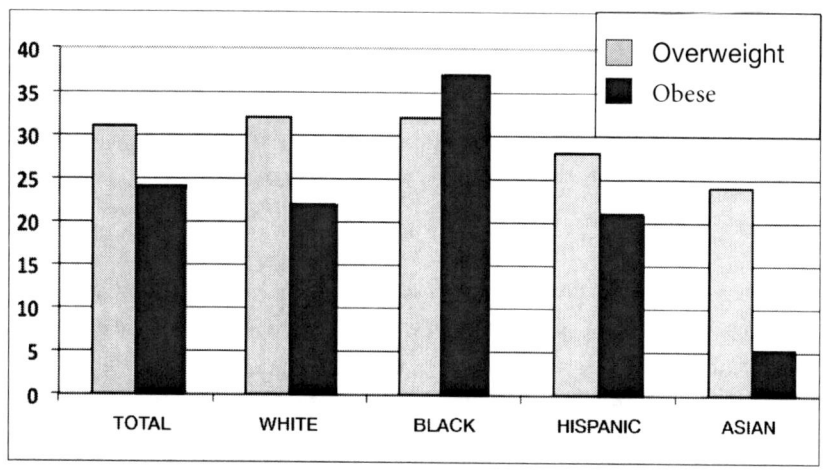

Chart 2. Percentage of adults 18 to 64 who are overweight or obese. The Commonwealth Fund.[4]

THE NEW FOOD RULES

Is this you? Coffee on an empty stomach, skipping breakfast, going hours without food and consuming foods that lack nutritional density? In my health coaching practice, I see two reoccurring culprits among people with bad health habits. First, people are not eating for prolonged periods of time and secondly, when they do eat their choices lack nutrition. These bad habits alone will leave you overweight, fatigued, de-hydrated, less likely to succeed, grumpy and over time among the ranks of the chronically ill.

Is this really what you want?

If the answer is yes you will want to discontinue reading this book. However if you are looking for sustainable, measurable and affordable means to get healthy, stay healthy, lose weight, increase energy, gain self-esteem and be a blessing to the people you have been assigned to in the world continue reading this book. It is truly your lucky day.

Rule of thumb is if the foods you are eating do not grow in the earth, do not swim in the sea or does not have wings to fly or legs to walk, is not harvested or considered a grain, nut or seed you will want to consider what it is you are consuming. Now I am not trying to scare you but truth is what you eat should be plant, animal or at the very least should have lived at some point.

Have you ever seen a Cheetos tree? How about a soda pop farm?

To my vegan and vegetarian friends: although I will not go into the many benefits of this lifestyle choice, please see chapter 8 for vegan and vegetarian recipes.

Our bodies require whole foods. Foods that when consumed send a signal to every part of our bodies (organs, tissue, blood, brain, etc.) that something of value has just happened. The body likes the signals it is receiving and utilizes the food for every function imaginable from energy and digestion to great looking hair, skin, nails, teeth and mood.

SUGAR

Sugar is a sticky subject; it is addictive and hidden in just about everything we eat and drink. As a health coach educating people on what they are consuming is important to me. Understanding how we got where we are is helpful in making lifestyle changes. Let's look at the brief History of Sugar according to Wikipedia. Sugar has five phases:

1. The extraction of sugar cane juice from the sugar cane plant and the subsequent domestication of the plant in tropical Southeast Asia many thousands of years ago.

2. The invention of manufacturing cane sugar granules from the sugar cane juice in India a little over two thousand years ago, followed by improvements in refining the crystal granules in India in the early centuries A. D.

3. The spread of cultivation and manufacturing of cane sugar to the medieval Islamic world together with some improvements of production methods.

4. The spread of cultivation and manufacturing of cane sugar to the west indies and tropical parts of the Americas beginning in the 16th century, followed by more intensive improvements in production in the 17th – 19th centuries in that part of the world.

5. The development of beet sugar, high fructose corn syrup and other sweeteners in the 19th and 20th centuries.

In short high fructose corn syrup was rapidly introduced to many processed foods and soft drinks in the United States between 1975 and 1985.

High fructose corn syrup is derived from corn. Corn is a domestic crop in the United States and Canada thus making corn more economical. American farmers are also paid government subsidies to grow corn crop keeping the price low. Because of these factors high fructose corn syrup quickly became an attractive low cost sweetener in America.

In recent years studies have noted an increase in high fructose corn syrup linked to various health conditions, such as metabolic syndrome, hypertension, dyslipemia, hepatic steatosis, insulin resistance, and obesity.

Broken down into simplest terms there are two types of sugar; fructose and glucose.

Fructose is found in fruits and vegetables. Glucose is found in all major carbohydrates such as processed foods, table sugar and fruits and vegetables. The glucose in the fruits and vegetables are natural sugars and provide the body with many benefits, however too much glucose can be detrimental to your health.

Both fructose and glucose provide good sources of energy and satisfy a sweet tooth. However excessive amounts of either can be fatal.

WHAT DIABETICS NEED TO KNOW

Diabetes is a disease. I hesitate to say chronic disease because so many with Type 2 diabetes have shown how a balanced mind set, proper nutrition and physical activity can create favorable management of diabetes and even eliminate symptoms all together. There are three different types of diabetes. Type 1 is where the body does not make insulin. Insulin helps get blood sugar into the body's cells and gives them energy. People with Type 1 diabetes should take daily insulin. Type 2 diabetes is where the body does not make enough insulin or use insulin well. This type of diabetes maybe treated with pills or shots, diet and activity. Pre-diabetes is when blood sugar levels are higher than normal but not high enough to have diabetes. People with pre-diabetes have a higher chance for Type 2 diabetes, heart disease and stroke.

DIABETES AND YOUR BODY

Diabetes changes the way your body uses food for energy, causing high blood pressure, which in turn acts like a slow processing poison to the body. According to studies conducted at the Mayo Clinic, high sugar levels slowly erode the ability of cells in the pancreas to make insulin. The pancreas over compensates and insulin levels remain overly high. Gradually, the pancreas is permanently damaged. All the excess sugar is modified in the blood. The elevated sugar in the blood causes changes that lead to Atherosclerosis, a hardening of the blood vessel. High sugar levels can lead to damage anywhere in the body. Damage to blood vessels, in particular, means no area is safe from too much sugar. High sugar levels and damaged blood vessels cause a multitude of complications that can come with diabetes such as:

- Kidney failure/disease, including dialysis
- Strokes & Heart attacks
- Vision problems, including blindness
- Immune Suppression
- Erectile Dysfunction
- Neuropathy
- Poor circulation
- Poor wound healing, in extreme cases; possible amputation

Is this what you want?

It is important to know your numbers. Normal range for fasting blood glucose levels is 70-99. Non fasting glucose levels range from 70-119. For Diabetics normal range for fasting blood glucose levels is 70 – 130. For Diabetics non-fasting glucose levels should be less than 180 after a meal.

What's Food Got To Do With It?

Alternative Forms of Sweeteners

LIQUID SWEETENERS

Agave Nectar - is naturally extracted from a cactus-like plant native to Mexico. All agave nectars dissolve easily.

Barley Malt Syrup - is made from soaking and sprouting barley and cooking down into the starch converts into sugar comes in liquid and powder form.

Organic Blackstrap Molasses - is a thick with a deep rich flavor molasses is rich in iron and other minerals.

Organic Raw Honey – Honey has been used around the world and has many health benefits. To get maximum benefits from honey make sure it is organic and raw. Honey can be used on just about anything.

Sorghum - from the sweet sorghum plant, the taste is similar to molasses. The juice is extracted from the plant and then boiled down to syrup.

Yacon - especially beneficial for those with high blood sugar works as a prebiotic and is great for digestive health.

GRANULATED SWEETENERS

Amasake – Native to Japan this is an ancient whole grain sweetener is made from cultured brown rice and is widely known for its healing properties.

Whole Cane Sugar - AKA Dried Cane Juice is made from the dried juice of the sugar cane plant and is similar to brown sugar with less sweetness.

Coconut Palm Sugar – AKA Coconut Nectar Sugar or Coconut Sugar is naturally sweet and nutrient-rich. This sweetener is a friendly choice for diabetics.

Date Sugar - made from ground dehydrated dates similar to brown sugar in taste with less sweetness. Granules do not dissolve in liquid and contains some gluten.

Lucuma – is made from an exotic fruit known as the "Gold of the Inca." This sweetener is diabetic friendly and widely known for its healing properties. Has a creamy taste similar to maple.

Maple Sugar - the sap of the sugar maple is boiled for longer than is needed to create maple syrup. After boiling a solid sugar remains.

Organic Sugar - comes from sugar cane grown free of chemicals or pesticides. It contains molasses and is darker than white sugar.

Turbinado - AKA Raw Sugar but it's not actually raw. It is processed but a better choice than white table sugar.

OTHER SWEETENERS

Maltitol, Maltitol Syrup, Sorbitol, Mannitol, Xylitol, Lactitol, Isomalt - these sugar alcohols naturally occur in plants, but are usually manufactured from sugars and starches. with fewer calories than sugars because the body can not completely absorb this can cause fermentation in the intestines that lead to gas, bloating and diarrhea.

Stevia - is derived from the leaves of a South American shrub, *Stevia rebaudiana*. Stevia is sweeter than cane sugar. Stevia is calorie free as it is not absorbed through the digestive tract. Stevia does not affect blood sugar levels and is diabetic friendly and can be purchased as a dried leaf, liquid extract, or powder.

FAKE FOODS

In my health coaching practice the rule of thumb is that if it does not grow on a tree, in the ground or at some point has not crawled, swam or walked then you should not be eating it. In simple terms, if it is not a plant or animal, it is most likely refined and processed which makes it a fake food.

The truth is fake foods are convenient and cheap. Today, you can grab a bag of chips and a soda pop for breakfast for about three bucks or a fast food breakfast sandwich for about one dollar. Do you really want the things you put into your body to be quick and cheap? When you eat like that please do not be deceived. You are in essence writing your own

What's Food Got To Do With It?

personal prescription to becoming overweight over time grumpy and chronically ill.

Studies show that roughly 70% of the Standard American Diet (SAD) is made up of fake foods. Plain and simple there are ways to eat healthy and save money in the process. Chapter 7 offers step by step directions on how and what to consume to eat healthy and be healthy.

Think of your body as a machine with an on/off switch. Every time you eat fruits, vegetables and quality grains and proteins, the body's switch automatically activates welcoming all the nutrients into the body to use and store for later. The body is happy that you were so thoughtful it processes the good skipping down the street whistling, singing and smiling knowing that you, its master, will treat it kindly again and takes great comfort in that.

On the other hand, put into the body fake foods and the body never has a chance to activate its on switch. Your body is in the off position constantly in defense mode attempting first to figure out what you have done and then working hard to rid itself of the self inflicted invasion that you, its master, has orchestrated. The fake foods body is always tired, overwhelmed, nutritionally underpaid and in a dead end situation. This body is sad and it walks down the street with its head down, lackluster and hardly smiling. Is this really how you planned on caring for your body?

Most Popular Fake Foods and What to Replace Them With

Bad Snack	Good Snack
Potato chips	Fresh veggie medley with dressing dip
Fried French fries	Olive oil baked French fries or sweet potato fries with sea salt
Candy	Homemade Trail mix Sesame, cranberry, dark choc, walnuts, cashew
Pastries (Cookies, doughnuts, pies, cakes)	Fresh fruit and sunflower seeds
Ice cream, JELLO, and puddings	Berries, Nuts, Greek yogurt, and Gelato
Bad Drinks	**Good Drinks**
Soda pop	Water infused with cucumber, ginger, and mint
Sweet tea	Green tea with lemon
Fruit juices	100% Fruit juices (Diluted with green tea, water, or vegetable juice)
Energy drinks	Naturally juiced fruits and vegetables and smoothies
Coffee drinks	Teas, water, and vegetable juices

Keep in mind you can still have some of the things on the left side of the list on occasion. It's not about taking everything away; it's about bringing balance to food and life.

ALOCHOL

Every generation has had its choice of alcohol. You may remember back in the day when Boones Farm, Brass Monkey and Colt 45 where popular cocktails. Today, the variety of alcohol available to us has grown. Alcohol is much more complicated and expensive than ever before in history with specialty cocktails like jumbo margaritas, cosmos and beers from around the globe. It is clear that in many communities alcohol has become more sophisticated as our diets continue to lag behind.

If you are indulging in spirits, I realize that what I say here today may not stop you. However, I advise you to pick your poison. Decide that you will incorporate healthy eating and some form of exercise into your weekly schedule. This way when it comes time to turn up you have some nutritional equity built in.

WINE, WATER & WHISKEY

At public speaking engagements one of the questions I ask my audiences is what does wine, water and whiskey have in common? The answer is they can all kill you if you have too much. So for all my wine heads let me dispel the myth that you can have wine often. Please know that over consumption of wine is no better for you than over consumption of hard liquor or water.

Some years ago someone in the medical community announced that wine is good for you. People armed with half the facts took that information and used it as a way to consume more of this spirit guilt free. The truth about wine is that it contains a chemical called resveratrol that studies have shown to, in moderation, benefit heart health.

According to the Mayo Clinic red wine, in moderation, has long been thought of as heart-healthy. The alcohol and certain substances in red wine called antioxidants may help prevent heart disease by increasing levels of high density lipoprotein (HDL) cholesterol (the good cholesterol) and protecting against artery damage.

While the news about red wine might sound great, if you enjoy a glass of red wine with your evening meal, doctors are weary of encouraging anyone to start drinking alcohol. That is because too much alcohol can have many harmful effects on your body.

Still, many doctors agree that something in red wine appears to help your heart. It is possible that antioxidants, such as flavonoids or a substance called resveratrol, have heart-healthy benefits.

Red wine seems to have even more heart-healthy benefits than do other types of alcohol, but it is possible that red wine is not any better than beer, white wine or hard liquor for heart health. There is still no clear evidence that red wine is better than other forms of alcohol when it comes to possible heart-healthy benefits.

Antioxidants in red wine called polyphenols may help protect the lining of blood vessels in your heart. Resveratrol in red wine might be a key ingredient that helps prevent damage to blood vessels, reduces low-density lipoprotein (LDL) cholesterol ("bad" cholesterol) and prevents blood clots.

Most research on resveratrol has been done on animals, not people. Research in mice given resveratrol suggests that the antioxidant might also help protect them from obesity and diabetes, both of which are strong risk factors for heart disease. However, those findings were reported only in mice, not in people. In addition, to get the same dose of resveratrol used in the mice studies, a person would have to drink more than 1,000 liters of red wine every day. Research in pigs has shown that resveratrol may improve heart function and increase the body's ability to use insulin. Again, however, these benefits have not been tested on people.

Some research shows resveratrol could be linked to a reduced risk of inflammation and blood clotting, both of which can lead to heart disease. More research is needed before it is known whether resveratrol was the cause for the reduced risk. However, one study showed that resveratrol may actually reduce the positive effects of exercise on the heart in older men. It is also important to know that resveratrol's effects only last a short time after drinking red wine, so its effects may not be long term.

The resveratrol in red wine comes from the skin of grapes used to make wine. Because red wine is fermented with grape skins longer than is white wine, red wine contains more resveratrol. Simply eating grapes, or drinking grape juice, has been suggested as one way to get resveratrol without drinking alcohol. Red and purple grape juices may have some of the same heart-healthy benefits of red wine.

Other foods containing some resveratrol include peanuts, blueberries and cranberries. It is not yet known how beneficial eating grapes or other foods might be compared with drinking red wine when it comes to promoting heart health. The amount of resveratrol in food and red wine can vary widely.

Resveratrol supplements also are available. While researchers have not found any harm in taking resveratrol supplements, most of the resveratrol in the supplements cannot be absorbed by your body.

Various studies have shown that moderate amounts of all types of alcohol benefit your heart, not just alcohol found in red wine. It is thought that alcohol:

- Raises high-density lipoprotein (HDL) cholesterol, the "good" cholesterol
- Reduces the formation of blood clots
- Helps prevent artery damage caused by high levels of low-density lipoprotein (LDL) cholesterol, the "bad" cholesterol
- Produces changes in blood pressure

Red wine's potential heart-healthy benefits look promising. Those who drink moderate amounts of alcohol, including red wine, seem to have a lower risk of heart disease. However, more research is needed before we know whether red wine is better for your heart than are other forms of alcohol, such as beer or spirits.

Neither the American Heart Association, nor the National Heart, Lung, and Blood Institute recommend that you start drinking alcohol just to prevent heart disease. Alcohol can be addictive and can cause or worsen other health problems.

Drinking too much alcohol increases your risk of high blood pressure, high triglycerides, liver damage, obesity, certain types of cancer, accidents and other problems. In addition, drinking too much alcohol regularly can cause weakened heart muscle (cardiomyopathy), leading to symptoms of heart failure in some people. If you have heart failure or a weak heart, you should avoid alcohol completely. If you take aspirin daily, you should avoid or limit alcohol, depending on your doctor's advice. You also should not drink alcohol if you are pregnant. If you have questions about the benefits and risks of alcohol, talk to your doctor about specific recommendations for you.

If you already drink red wine, do so in moderation. For healthy adults, that means up to one drink a day for women of all ages and men older than age 65, and up to two drinks a day for men age 65 and younger. The limit for men is higher because men generally weigh more and have more of an enzyme that metabolizes alcohol than women do.

A drink is defined as 12 ounces (355 milliliters, or mL) of beer, 5 ounces (148 mL) of wine or 1.5 ounces (44 mL) of 80-proof distilled spirits.

Foods with Resveratrol & Antioxidants	Contains
Red Grapes	Manganese, potassium and vitamins K, C and B1
Peanut Butter	Niacin and Manganese
Dark Chocolate	Antioxidants, minerals iron, copper and manganese.
Blueberries	Antioxidants, dietary fiber, vitamins C and K and manganese.

TOBACCO

Let's just get this out the way; I have smoked over the years from time to time. I was never a heavy smoker (less than a pack per week) just enough to kill me. Mostly I smoked socially as we all know how great a cigarette is with your morning coffee break or at happy hour after the first cocktail. I do not judge. I know quitting is a real struggle and anyone can get caught up in this addiction because of its habit forming effects.

Tobacco is a cousin to alcohol and caffeine. Anyone who has ever smoked knows that where there is alcohol or caffeine tobacco is not usually far behind.

If you are a smoker you should look at smoking as a food source, in fact most people consume cigarettes for breakfast, lunch and dinner. After all smokers put cigarettes up to their mouths, you inhale them along with the tobacco, nicotine and 500 other carcinogenics that enter the body to nourish it with poison. Remember everything you put in your body either helps or hurts.

Let's be honest with each other. Most smokers are not eating their peas and carrots and doing pushups between smoke breaks. In fact, for many smokers smoking represents breakfast along with a nice sugary beverage. Once again lunch is fake fast food accompanied by a smoke and everyone has heard of the after dinner drink and smoke. Bottom line folks this is a whole lot of nothing for the body to attempt to sort out day after day.

What's Food Got To Do With It?

A BRIEF HISTORY OF TABACCO

Tobacco was used by pre Columbian Americans. Later Native Americans cultivated the plant and smoked it in pipes for medicinal and ceremonial purposes. In the mid 16th century Europe began to popularize its use with France, Portugal, Spain and England.

By 1612 the first successful crop was cultivated in Virginia within seven years tobacco became the colony's largest export. Over the next two centuries, the growth of tobacco as a cash crop fueled the demand in North America for slave labor.

COACH KENYA ON TABACCO

It used to be that as the price of cigarettes skyrocketed people stopped smoking. Then big tobacco got smart creating less expensive versions of the more popular cigarettes so that everyone could afford a little cancer and heart disease. Minority communities played right into the hands of big tobacco. Not to mention that marketing by cigarette companies (BIG TABACCO) is very aggressive in poor and minority neighborhoods such as is that for alcohol and fast food. Companies know that poor people and minorities may not be able to afford a trip to Europe but they can sure run down to the corner store and grab a pack of cigarettes, a pop and some chips. In many poorer communities a new trend has emerged. Demand has been created for cigar type products like BLACK and MILD due to their low cost. The problem is people are smoking more of these cigar type products creating a new catastrophic health hazard from smoking. Another trend is the sell of loose cigarettes allowing people to purchase just a few cigarettes at a time at a fraction of what it would cost to purchase an entire pack. This trend has its pros and cons as most people who purchase this way are cutting back on their daily consumption. However if this method where not available possibly they would have quit smoking all together due to the skyrocketing cost of cigarettes. This method is illegal and measuring its effects has not yet been determined.

According to the American Lung Association's website (www.lung.org), there are approximately 600 ingredients in cigarettes when burned, they create more than 7,000 chemicals at least 69 of these chemicals are known to cause cancer, and many are poisonous.

CHEMICALS IN TOBACCO SMOKE AND OTHER PLACES THEY ARE FOUND
Acetone – found in nail polish remover
Acetic Acid – an ingredient in hair dye
Ammonia – a common household cleaner
Arsenic – used in rat poison
Benzene – found in rubber cement
Butane – used in lighter fluid
Cadmium – active component in battery acid
Carbon Monoxide – released in car exhaust fumes
Formaldehyde – embalming fluid
Hexamine – found in barbecue lighter fluid
Lead – used in batteries
Napthalene – an ingredient in moth balls
Methanol – a main component in rocket fuel
Nicotine – used as insecticide
Tar – material for paving roads
Toluene - used to manufacture paint

Table 1. Chemicals in tobacco smoke and where they are found. American Lung Association.[5]

For help with smoking cessation go to www.lung.org or contact your local health provider.

A BREIF HISTORY OF CAFFIENE

Caffeine is one of the world's most widely used drugs and largely associated with coffee. Coffee originated in Ethiopia and was later introduced to Arabia and the rest of the east. In 1573, coffee was introduced to the Europeans. Tea was later introduced around 1657 and became very popular among Europeans. Near the end of the 19th century cola products started to emerge around the world and became one of the more popularized caffeine drinks. So popular that Coca Cola replaced cocaine for sugar and caffeine in its formula, shortly after the FDA filed a lawsuit to remove caffeine from Coca Cola. The lawsuit was successful in reducing the amount of caffeine in Coke.

COACH KENYA'S CAFFIENE STORY

The subject of caffeine is part two of my confession. As a kid, I swore I would never touch the stuff. Coffee was the furthest thing from my mind. In fact, the smell of it nauseated me. Soda pop on the other hand was my beverage of choice; there was nothing like a bag of hot stuff potato chips and an RC cola pop. I did not drink nearly the amount of pop as most kids in my neighborhood because my mama was semi health conscious about what we ate and drank but that certainly did not stop me from hitting the corner store when I had an extra twenty five cents. In my teen age years I became more conscious of my weight and pop had been exchanged for more sophisticated beverages. It was not until college that I became a coffee drinker. Many of my peers counted on coffee as a pick me upper so naturally I tried the popular concoction – heavy cream, heavy sugar. I immediately noticed the weight gain and rise and fall in energy I experienced when I drank coffee. I attribute this awareness to the fact that I was more in touch than the average person regarding how my body felt when introduced to new foods due to years of paying attention to my body by managing my weight.

Fast forward 25 years later coffee is my hero and a true friend in my time of need. It is always available and always hits the spot. I am proud to say that I am a one cup (14oz) per day drinker and I never became one of those coffee all day people that drank coffee in lieu of meals but in my one cup per day quest I know coffee is my guilty caffeine pleasure.

Since then I have graduated to Starbucks, the queen of coffee. I continue to be a one cup per day drinker, but never on an empty stomach and always with a large water chaser. I cannot quite brag that I drink black coffee but I am proud to say that my coffee contains minuscule amounts of sugars and cream. From time to time I will go a few days without coffee to play a game with myself to overcome the daily addiction. I believe anything you must have daily, with the exception of the love of God, you should refrain from for a bit to remind yourself that you are in control of what you eat, think and do.

The bottom line is that caffeine in any form is a stimulant. Think about the things that you put into your body that instantly change your mood; chocolate, marijuana, drugs, alcohol and caffeine. Studies show that moderate uses of caffeine have some benefits.

As a practicing Health Coach, I advise my clients to listen to their bodies. The number one expert on you is you. If you are consuming caffeine on a regular basis meaning you have to have it every day, think about whether your consumption has become an addiction. If you are a one cup a day coffee drinker, take a few days off just to show caffeine who is in charge. If you are that person that drinks caffeine products all throughout the day you will want to reevaluate your relationship.

Here's a chart of some common caffeine sources and exactly how much of a wallop each packs:

Caffeine Sources	Approximate Caffeine Content (mg)
Coffee, regular (1 cup)	138
Espresso (1/4 cup)	125
Cappuccino, regular (1 cup)	60
Latte, regular (1 cup)	60
Tea, brewed, hot (1 cup)	47
Nestea Iced Tea, Earl Grey (1 cup)	33
Cola soda, regular or diet (12 oz)	42
Mountain Dew (12 oz)	52
Chocolate, semisweet (1 oz)	18
Chocolate milk (1 cup)	5
Cocoa powder (1 tablespoon)	12

Table 2. Healthier sources of caffeine. WebMD.[6]

LACK OF INTIMACY

Sex is everywhere but intimacy you will have to look deep for. During an interview with Oprah, Jane Fonda admitted she had married several times before she had experienced a sense of intimacy.

"Perhaps you think that by intimacy I mean sex, so allow me to clarify. Sex can be intimate but is not necessarily so; sometimes it is just a pleasurable stimulation of genitalia. By intimacy I mean an attunement between two people who, despite each other's evident flaws, open their hearts fully to each other. This openness makes them vulnerable. So trust is key. So is self – love: it is impossible to be truly intimate with someone if you do not like yourself."

~Jane Fonda, My Life So Far

People crave intimacy. I know I do. I am not just talking about that boy meets girl type of intimacy it goes much deeper than that. I am speaking of an intimacy between a parent and child or the desire to have a friend that you can share life's moments with. I can remember growing up when people would walk past one another and make eye contact perhaps say "what's up doc" or just give a simple head nod to acknowledge that you see them. In the fast pace society we live in even simple gestures like that have vanished. Folks are not paying attention to themselves and their own wants and needs let alone being focused on yours. That is the bad news. The good news is people want connections (intimacy) with other people. We have simply gotten away from where intimacy comes from. Many are reaching for a false sense of intimacy in the form of money, cars, clothes, food, casual relationships and even drugs and alcohol to make them feel.

COACH KENYA'S RECOMMENDATIONS FOR INTIMACY

Blaise Pascal a French mathematician, physicist, inventor, writer and Christian philosopher stated that all of humanity's problems stem from man's inability to sit quietly in a room alone. No truer statement has been made. I am not sure how practical sitting quietly in a room would be with the pace of today's hectic society. But here are a few simple things you can practice daily to bring your thoughts into balance and encourage intimacy with yourself and others.

- Practicing intimacy with you; breathing, hot baths, hot towel massage, professional message, workout, walk, music, meditation and reading.
- Practicing intimacy with others; hugs, eye contact, being soft spoken, sitting quietly, reading, walking, healthy meals, and board games.
- I encourage you to steal moments as often as possible until these practices become a habit.

TESTIMONIAL

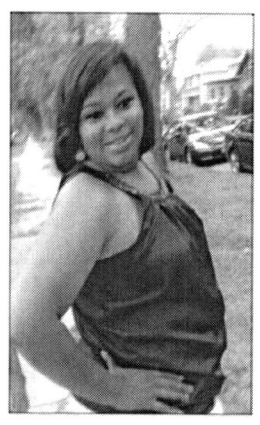

Andrea Newton, Chicago, IL
BODY DIVINE WEIGHT LOSS CLIENT

Challenge - inflammation, weight Loss

Personal Questionnaire

Q. What results have you achieved (i.e. weight loss, inches, medical, personal)?

R. I have reached results that I could not have achieved on my own. I am no longer at risk for high blood pressure, stroke, or diabetes. I have been diagnosed with carpal tunnel and tendonitis but I have discovered what to eat that will prevent the diseases from flaring up.

When I started I had problems with (food choices, diabetes, weight, sleep, mood). I had problems about being uneducated about food choices now I am more aware of what types of food provide the best health for me. I also learned I needed to have a coach that was willing to go the distance with me; I could not have done this on my own.

Q. Where were you before starting BODY DIVINE?

Before starting BODY DIVINE, I was in a place mentally where I had given up.

Q. What has been your biggest achievement thus far in the program? Name more than one, if applicable.

R. My biggest achievement is I am no longer considered a risk for high blood pressure and diabetes. Another achievement is that I have learned through trial and error with my coach that the food choices I make will determine if I have flare ups.

Q. Where are you now?

R. I went from a size 16W (I refused to wear 18) currently I am in a loose fitting 14 on my way to a size 12. So thank you Kenya for turning my life around for the better. Oh my son says thank you for helping to extend he's mother's life.

Coach's Comments...

Andrea and her husband joined the program with his diabetic health in mind. Andrea was clear that she did not like exercise and was not that interested in eating right. After weeks of consistency Andrea's entire demeanor changed and the favorable results followed. We made it through many setbacks. As a Coach I'd like to see all my clients make a touchdown and Andrea is well on her way to achieving a healthier lifestyle.

*And the day came
when the risk it took
to remain tight and closed in the bud
was more painful
than the risk it took to bloom.*[7]

-Alicia Keys

CHAPTER 3

Preventing Chronic Illness

Thus far we have talked in much detail about fake foods, sugar, alcohol, caffeine and relationships. Now let's bring it all together. What we are putting in our bodies and how we are spending our time is causing chronic illness and premature death. And in between the time it takes chronic illness to manifest poor food choices are causing Americans to be overweight, obese, grumpy, impotent, unemployable, disable and broke with an inability to create and sustain viable relationships with ourselves, one another and the communities we are responsible for serving.

Houston, we got a problem.

The good news is there is a doable solution.

A big part of the solution is nutrition through quality primary and secondary food. One common denominator between all that ails us is food. The past few years I have lived in my native city of Chicago. The news has been plagued with violence, shootings and death. The truth is this curse has not displayed itself everywhere in the city just certain neighborhoods. The neighborhoods are minority, low income neighborhoods that lack opportunity and yes are undernourished in many ways. I do not personally know the shooters that perpetuated these crimes but I am willing to bet that the shooters are not surrounded by loving relationships, eating salmon, broccoli and quinoa and practicing self-care on a daily basis.

Certain things equal certain things. When you practice poor nutrition you will project poor energy around you. Likewise when you practice proper nutrition and self-care that energy too will project around everyone in its path. In other words a diet filled with missed meals, caffeine, sugar, alcohol, nicotine and no nutrition produces a person that is high strung yet lazy, lacks creativity yet is aggressive, moody and angry. When you take these ingredients and add poverty, toxic relationships, unemployment, lack of opportunity and guns – You produce a shooter.

In contrast add the opposite ingredients to a person's existence such as opportunity, good relationships, proper nutrition and self-care and you will get quite a different set of results.

COACH KENYA'S RECOMMENDATION ON PREVENTION

With myriads of information floating around it becomes overwhelming as to where to start. I recommend you begin with the smallest most doable step, nutrition. Let's face it, it takes time to climb out of poverty, create jobs and build great relationships but nutrition and self-care start at your very next meal. Once you practice your own personal self-care plan you will begin to not only energize yourself but those around you creating a domino effect. Practice these principles time and time again and things will begin to turn. When thoughts change about what you deserve actions soon follow. Back up and put it in reverse for those of you that are not quite convinced. Let's approach the issue from a different angle: Ask yourself how did I get where I am? Whatever your circumstance how did I get here? Keep going full throttle with the good that you are doing. The areas that are not working consider doing the opposite of what got you where you are. For example if you are overweight from not eating, not drinking water and making poor food choices when you eat, then try the reverse, eat more frequent meals, drink eight glasses of water daily and when you eat make healthy choices. I would like to take credit for all the positive changes you will experience over time but the truth is it is not rocket science. It is simply the way the body works. It is what has gotten us into this mess and what will get us out.

For the many reading this book you either provide support to someone chronically ill or have a chronic condition you are looking to manage. First understand you are not alone. As of 2012, about half of all adults over 100 million people have one or more chronic health conditions. One of four adults has two or more chronic health conditions and the number is on the rise. More importantly know that you are not your illness and that your body is a well designed creation that wants to work for you. If you are prescribed medicine please follow your Doctor's orders. Know that medicine is designed to work best with people who practice diets high in nutrition. If you are not following Doctors orders and practicing proper nutrition you are in essence digging a premature grave that will not only effect you but those around you for generations to come.

14 Healthy Habits of Successful People
Actively practices self-care
Avoids junk foods in the home
Drinks plenty of water daily
Eats whole foods with each meal
Eats a minimum of three meals per day
Engages in optimistic relationships and conversations
Has a vision for the future
Keeps healthy snacks available
Knows how to manage stress, anxiety and worry
Looks for the beauty in every situation
Practices deep breathing
Practices excellence in all things
Practices a regular sleep schedule
Takes time out for physical activity & fun

Your body is a temple,
but only if you treat it as one. [8]

    —Astrid Alauda

CHAPTER 4

Food As Medicine

THE NUTRIENTS YOU NEED TO KNOW

By now you have heard the terms nutrition and nutritionally dense many times but what do these terms really mean? You have also been introduced to the theory of primary foods (relationships) and secondary foods (foods you eat).

When it comes to secondary foods, the foods you eat, the body needs certain nutrients to thrive. These nutrients are referred to as macro nutrients and micro nutrients.

Macro nutrients are carbohydrates, fiber, protein and fat. In everyday food language this would look like rice or sweet potato as carbohydrates, fish or steak as protein and avocado or olive oil as good fat. These nutrients provide the body with the big calories required for energy and basic function.

MACRONUTRIENTS

Carbohydrates are the macronutrients that we need in the largest amounts. According to the Dietary Reference Intakes published by the USDA, 45% - 65% of calories should come from carbs. We need this amount of carbohydrates because:

- Carbs are the body's main source of fuel.
- Carbs are easily used by the body for energy.
- All of the tissues and cells in our body can use glucose energy.
- Carbs are needed for the central nervous system, the kidneys, the brain, the muscles (including heart) to function properly.
- Carbs can be stored in the muscle and liver and later used for energy.
- Carbs are important for intestinal health and waste elimination.
- Carbs are mainly found in starchy foods (like grains and potatoes), fruit, milk and yogurt. Other foods like vegetables, beans, nuts, seeds, and cottage cheese contain carbohydrates, but in lesser amounts.

FIBER

Fiber refers to certain types of carbohydrates that our body cannot digest. These carbohydrates pass through the intestinal tract intact and help to move waste out of the body. Diets that are low in fiber have been shown to cause problems such as constipation and hemorrhoids and to increase the risk for certain types of cancer such as colon cancer. Diets high in fiber; however, have been shown to decrease the risk for heart disease, obesity, and help lower cholesterol. Foods high in fiber include fruits, vegetables, and whole grain products.

PROTEIN

According to the Dietary Reference Intakes published by the USDA 10% - 35% of calories should come from protein. Most Americans get plenty of protein, and easily meet this need by consuming a balanced diet. We need protein for:

- Growth (especially important for children, teens and pregnant women)
- Tissue repair
- Immune function
- Making essential hormones and enzymes
- Energy when carbs are not available
- Preserving lean muscle mass

Protein is found in meats, poultry, fish, meat substitutes, cheese, milk, nuts, legumes, and in smaller quantities in starchy foods and vegetables. When we eat these types of foods, our body breaks down the protein that they contain into amino acids (the building blocks of proteins). Some amino acids are essential which means that we need to get them from our diet, and others are non essential which means that our body can make them. Protein that comes from animal sources contains all of the essential amino acids that we need. Plant sources of protein, on the other hand, do not contain all of the essential amino acids.

FAT

Although fats have received a bad reputation for causing weight gain, some fat is essential for survival. According to the Dietary Reference Intakes published by the USDA 20% - 35% of calories should come from fat. We need this amount of fat for:

- Normal growth and development
- Energy (fat is the most concentrated source of energy)
- Absorbing certain vitamins (like A, D, E, K and carotenoids)
- Provide cushioning for organs
- Maintaining cell membranes
- Providing taste, consistency, and stability to foods

Fat is found in meat, poultry, nuts, milk products, butters and margarines, oils, lard, fish, grain products and salad dressings. There are three main types of fat: saturated fat, unsaturated fat, and trans fat. Saturated fat (is found in foods like meat, butter, lard, and cream) and trans fat (found in baked goods, snack foods, fried foods, and margarines) have been shown to increase your risk for heart disease. Replacing saturated and trans fat in your diet with unsaturated fat (found in foods like olive oil, avocados, nuts, and canola oil) has been shown to decrease the risk of developing heart disease.

Although macronutrients are very important they are not the only thing we need for survival. Our bodies also need water (6-8 glasses a day) and micronutrients. Micronutrients are nutrients that our bodies need in smaller amounts, and include vitamins and minerals.

MICRONUTRIENTS

Micro means small so the micronutrients are the nutrients that we need in small amounts. These include the 12 vitamins and 13 minerals that we need every day. Vitamins are categorized as water soluble or fat soluble depending on whether they can dissolve in fat or water. Minerals are divided into two groups, the major minerals and the trace minerals. They are available as dietary supplements but be careful not to go over the tolerable upper levels.

Water soluble vitamins include vitamin C and the seven B complex vitamins. They have a variety of functions and you need all of them to be healthy. Chronic deficiencies of these vitamins can result in poor health.

Fat soluble vitamins include vitamins A, D, E, and K. Vitamins A and E come strictly from the foods you eat. However your body can make both vitamin D and K. Your body can store these vitamins in fat tissue. While it is extremely difficult to get too much of these vitamins from the foods you eat, you can build up toxic amounts of these four vitamins if you take massive amounts as dietary supplements every day.

Major minerals include calcium, phosphorus, chloride, magnesium, potassium and sodium. These minerals are particularly important for healthy bones, teeth, muscle and fluid balance in the body. The trace minerals are chromium, copper, fluoride, iodine, iron, selenium and zinc. Your body needs all these minerals for a variety of processes to keep functioning.

PHYTONUTRIENTS

Phyto refers to plants. Many different phyto nutrients are found only in plants. Many of these natural chemicals are found in the colorful skins and flesh of fruits and vegetables. Some of the best known phyto nutrients are carotenoids, such as beta carotene, lutein, lycopene and zeaxanthin, plus flavonoids such as guercetin and anthocyanin. Phyto nutrients have a variety of functions in the body. Some of them may function as antioxidants that protect the cells in our bodies from free radical damage. Others, like falcarinol from carrots, may help to prevent cancer.It is not known exactly how many of these different phytonutrients we need, however a healthy diet including at least five servings of fruits and colorful vegetables everyday will supply your body with lots of phytonutrients.

COACH KENYA'S RECOMMENDATION ON HOW TO EAT HEALTHY ON A BUDGET

It costs too much to eat healthy. I hear these words all the time. The truth is this statement is false and many people simply do not know how to accomplish eating healthy on a budget. In this section we will show you exactly what to do to accomplish these two goals with ease. First you must know that healthy foods such as fruits and vegetables cost a fraction of what their unhealthy counterparts (processed foods and fast foods) cost. In making this statement I will acknowledge that there are places referred to as food deserts where a single banana can cost $1.29. With ridiculous pricing like that most people if given the option between spending a buck on a single banana or a burger would pick the burger most often. However know that this is the exception to the rule and eating healthy costs less for those who are willing to prepare. If you are willing to make weekly trips to the grocery store for fresh produce I will show you how to eat healthy on a budget and save time and money to boot.

Go ahead and test my theory, on your next trip to the supermarket I want you to do one thing different. If you hardly every purchase fresh produce or purchase very little fresh produce I would like for you to up the ante and buy just a little bit more fresh produce than normal. Do not buy too much I would hate for it to spoil. Purchase only what you would consume in a week. Once you get to the checkout counter place all your fresh produce on the counter to be rung up first and check the total before the other items are calculated. Then add the meats, dairy, drinks, processed foods and anything that is not fresh produce. You are likely to see your bill triple or even quadruple right before your very eyes. This alone may be motivation enough to eat your vegetables.

The key to eating healthy on a budget is shopping and preparing your food at home. The cool thing about fresh produce (fruits and vegetables) is that they require little or no preparation as God in his infinite wisdom did the work for us. I'm thinking he knew what was best for our bodies.

  I have supplied a week's grocery list for you below and a three step guide to help you on your way to eating healthy, losing weight, saving money and most importantly fighting against chronic illness. It is highly recommended that you look into securing a Health Coach. Google Health Coaches in your area for a complete listing. If budget is a factor partner up with an accountability partner someone you spend an ample amount of time with each week like a spouse, co worker or friend.

THE EXACTLY WHAT TO EAT CHART

Pick a week's worth from each category. Remember your plate should contain **50% - 60% veggies – 10%-15% fruit 10% nuts or seeds & 20% animal proteins.**

VEGETABLES	**FRUIT**	Peanut butter
Fresh Salad Greens	Apple	Mixed nuts
-Spinach	Banana	Walnuts
- Cabbage	Blueberries	Peanuts
-Broccoli coleslaw	Strawberries	Almonds
-Swiss Chard	Raspberries	Sunflower seeds
-Arugula	Blackberries	Pumpkin seeds
-Romaine	Pineapple	Sesame seeds
Artichoke	Grapefruit	**PROTEIN**
Mung sprouts	**NUTS, SEEDS & FAT**	Eggs
Snow peas	Real Butter	Red snapper
Spinach	Olive oil	Perch
Collards	Coconut oil	Tilapia
Turnips	Sesame oil	Salmon
Mustard	*Cream cheese	Tuna
Celery	*Mayo	Mahi Mahi
Okra	*Sour cream	Cod
Asparagus	Avocado	Sardines
Cucumbers	Hummus	Chicken
String beans	Olives	Turkey
Broccoli	100% whole flaxseed	Turkey breakfast sausage
Squash	Natural cheese(s)	*Bacon
Cauliflower	Almond butter	Shrimp

What's Food Got To Do With It?

THE EXACTLY WHAT TO EAT CHART

Pick a week's worth from each category. Remember your plate should contain 50% - 60% veggies – 10%-15% fruit 10% nuts or seeds & 20% animal proteins.

Crab	Horseradish	**DRESSINGS**
Lobster	Vanilla	Ranch
Lamb	Jasmine	Oil & Vinegar
*Pork	Basil	Blue cheese
Ground turkey	Jasmine	Cesar
*Beef	Sage	Green Goddess
HERBS & SPICES		Balsamic vinaigrette
Fenugreek	**DRINKS**	
Bay leaf	Water	*coffee
Caraway	*Tea (Sweet, Regular)	*diet colas
Dill	Decaf Tea Bags green/white/reg.	*sugar free drink mix (any flavor)

*consume only on occasion as has low nutritional density

As a practicing Health Coach I hate to place restrictions on foods. However here are a few foods you will want to avoid or minimize. If you must have these foods always eat them as part of a balanced plate as they impact blood sugar when eaten alone: carrots, potatoes, peas, white rice, white pasta, corn, chips, sugar, sugary drinks, salt, flour, white bread, bagels and pastries.

Step 1 – SHOP

Make a list and go shopping. Do not overdo it! Grab a week's worth of groceries and remember to focus on vegetables and some fruits as your primary source of nutrients. Weigh yourself before you start. You will be astonished at the transformation in a short period of time.

Step 2 – PREP

Prepare an assortment of raw and cooked produce. Prepare enough for three to four days and throw it in a zip lock bag. Do not over complicate things, remember God already did the work. Your job is to have fun with different combinations of food. The key is to have them handy.

Step 3 – EAT

Get in three square meals each day! And yes, it is important to eat breakfast and break the fast. This does not mean you have to step out of bed and eat but by all means make every attempt to eat something at least an hour after waking.

Believe it or not this is where a lot of people fail. In my Health Coaching practice many clients come to me overweight and unhealthy because they do not eat breakfast, do not eat often enough and of course make poor food choices. If you can follow these three steps consistently over a 90 day period you will see tremendous changes in your health, mood and waistline (usually in the first 30 days). As you make your transformation do not forget to follow me on social media and share your experience.

What's Food Got To Do With It?

TESTIMONIAL

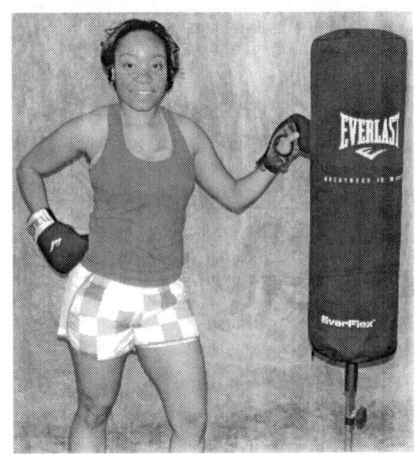

Shaleece Raymond
BODY DIVINE WEIGHT LOSS CLIENT

Challenge – eating healthy, weight loss

Personal Questionnaire

Q. *What results have you achieved (i.e. weight loss, inches, medical, personal)?*

R. *I am at the end of my first six week session and I have managed to lose over 10 pounds and 22.75 inches.*

When I started I had problems with (food choices, diabetes, weight, sleep, and mood)?

I have problems with food choices and mood; it was something I had adjusted to. I was also concerned about losing weight and putting it back on. I have been on many diets and BODY DIVINE has taught me how my body works.

Q. Where were you before starting BODY DIVINE?

R. I started at a weight 155 pounds. I thought I was eating right I had yogurt and all kinds of health snacks but did not shed a pound. Now I am losing weight and inches like crazy and I feel full of energy.

Q. What has been your biggest achievement thus far in the program? Name more than one, if applicable.

R. Losing weight, portion control, eating healthier, learning recipes, cooking more, and not giving up.

Q. Where are you now?

R. Currently I have reached my goal of 135 pounds and I have lost close to 40 inches over my entire body. I am amazed at how I look. I would encourage anyone to invest in themselves.

Coach's Comments...

I refer to Shaleece as my 20 pounder. Shaleece was a model client; she followed the program and rarely got off track. When she did fall off, she jumped right back on track. I attribute two key behaviors to Shaleece's success. First, her positive attitude and second her showing up. Shaleece has maintained her weight nicely. She will never have to worry about gaining weight again because her new eating and exercise habits are incorporated into her lifestyle. PS- Her husband is grateful, supportive and has expressed that he too has benefitted from the BODY DIVINE™ program.

*Tell me what you eat,
and I will tell you what you are.* [9]

-Jean Anthelme Brillat-Savarin

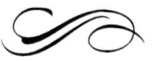

CHAPTER 5

Nutrition Anyone

COACH KENYA'S PERSONAL STORY

As a woman who has struggled with my weight and self-image my entire life, women's health is especially important to me. It started in grammar school when I noticed on school picture preview day that I was fat. I was happy but I was fat. I was cute but I was fat. As a child my mom did not allow lots of junk food into our home. I do remember salivating over my neighbor's food. Things like bacon, eggs, biscuits, tacos and plenty of pop and wanting to spend plenty of time over their houses to play and eat. The weird thing was that at that time my neighbors where not fat, I was. Later they would gain weight and develop food related illnesses. I went through many years of being teased or told I had a pretty face but… Because I was not the heaviest kid in school or in the neighborhood I spent my share of time name calling at those who weighed more than me. This was my way of taking the spotlight off of me. The truth was I was not comfortable in my own skin. By freshman year in high school I was still labeled as fat and still knew very little about proper nutrition. All I knew was I was eating much of the same things as my friends and they were not fat. I was determined to get the weight off and I did in all the wrong ways. I starved

What's Food Got To Do With It?

myself, I binged and purged, I took drugs and alcohol to suppress my appetite I even became a runner in an effort to lose the pounds. There were many points in which the weight came off only to return again. This battle would continue throughout my adult life including two pregnancies, two college degrees, two marriages, two divorces, many career changes, not to mention years in the gym.

How could one spend years in the gym and still be overweight? It was not until I made the personal connection between my body and the foods I ate that I was able to lose weight and truly connect with myself.

WOMEN'S NUTRITION

Whitney's dead ya'll and Bobby Brown is alive and doing quite well. Personally I am happy that Bobby is alive and well but still quite saddened when I think about the years taken off of Whitney's life. My point here is that women require very different nutrition than their male counterparts. All humans need the macro and micro nutrients I spoke about in chapter four to thrive and be well. When it comes to women and men there are real physical differences.

According to Dr. James Dobson's Family Talk, there are physical differences between men and women. Here are some physical characteristics unique to males and females. Men and women differ in countless ways, many of which they are not even conscious of. Here are just a few of those differences:

1) A woman has greater constitutional vitality, perhaps because of her unique chromosomal pattern. Normally, she outlives a man by three or four years in the U.S. Females simply have a stronger hold on life than males, even in the uterus. More than 140 male babies are conceived for every 100 females; by the time birth occurs, the ratio is 105 to 100, with the rest of the males dying in spontaneous abortions.
2) Men have a higher incidence of death from almost every disease except three: benign tumors, disorders related to female reproduction, and breast cancer.
3) Men have a higher rate of basal metabolism than women.

4) The sexes differ in skeletal structure, women having a shorter head, broader face, less protruding chin, shorter legs, and longer trunk. The first finger of a woman's hand is usually longer than the third; with men the reverse is true. Boys' teeth last longer than do those of girls.

5) Women have a larger stomach, kidneys, liver, and appendix, and smaller lungs than men.

6) Women have three very important physiological functions totally absent in men--menstruation, pregnancy, and lactation. Each of these mechanisms influences behavior and feelings significantly. Female hormonal patterns are more complex and varied. The glands work differently in the two sexes. For example, a woman's thyroid is larger and more active; it enlarges during menstruation and pregnancy, which makes her more prone to goiter, provides resistance to cold, and is associated with the smooth skin, relatively hairless body, and the thin layer of subcutaneous fat that are important elements in the concept of personal beauty. Women are also more responsive emotionally, laughing and crying more readily.

7) Women's blood contains more water (20 percent fewer red cells). Since red cells supply oxygen to the body, she tires more easily and is more prone to faint. Her constitutional viability is therefore strictly a long-range matter. When the working day in British factories, under wartime conditions, was increased from ten to twelve hours, accidents among women increased 150 percent; the rate of accidents among men did not increase significantly.

8) Men are 50 percent stronger than women in brute strength.

9) Women's hearts beat more rapidly than those of men (80 versus 72 beats per minute). Their blood pressure (ten points lower than men) varies more from minute to minute, but they have much less tendency to high blood pressure--at least until after menopause.

10) Female lung capacity is about 30 percent less than in males.

11) Women can withstand high temperatures better than men because their metabolism slows down less.

12) Men and women differ in every cell of their bodies because they carry a differing chromosomal pattern. The implications of those genetic components range from obvious to extremely subtle. For example, when researchers visited high school and college campuses to study behavior of the sexes, they observed that males and females even transported their books in different ways. The young men tended to carry them at their sides with their arms looped over the top. Women and girls, by

contrast, usually cradled their books at their breasts, in much the same way they would a baby.

MEN'S NUTRITION

Ladies this section is as much for you as for the men in your life. Men need a lot more than the big piece of chicken. Traditionally women are the caregivers of the family. Over the years this has changed and men have been left to fend for themselves. This is a bad move as we love our men and need them to live long and be healthy. Your man's health encourages your families health, your sexual pleasure and to some degree your financial fitness. So ladies, we really want to give our men more than the proverbial big piece of chicken.

From a health coaching perspective I can tell you that there is nothing worse than a Raggedy Ass Man (RAM) ok, maybe a Raggedy Ass Woman (RAW). Raggedy men cannot hear you much less nurture and care for you in the manner God intended. Even if they are good providers they likely have poor spending habits defeating the purpose of being a good provider. Additionally if you are not caring for yourself your are taking years off your life and your earning power.

My second marriage taught me a lot about health, finances and life in general. It amazed me that in the courtship phase of our relationship that my husband, by adopting my healthy habits, was able to drop over 70 pounds and discontinue medications he had relied on for years. While I gained over twenty pounds, lost my way and deteriorated my health by adopting just a few of his unhealthy habits. This might sound crazy but I personally thanked him for that experience although it ended in divorce. It was him that suggested I consider coaching, nutrition and fitness as a livelihood. It was also the bitterness of that divorce that taught me to protect my mind, body and money. Thanks darling!

The way to a man's health is through a woman. Women should be involved in their men's health for several reasons: they make the healthcare decisions in their families, women know the more about living a healthy lifestyle, and their health is directly connected to their mans health in many ways. In the past women have taken on the role of care giver for their family. They coordinate care of their children and sometimes their parents. It is women that spend on average eleven years out of the work forces caring for children and elderly parents they also do it for their husbands. Second, women know more about health than men and to be more active about prevention and treatment. Many women become experienced in care giving. However ladies if those two reasons don't exactly blown your skirt up here's a reason that might encourage you to get more involved in your man's health. Your health and well-being is connected to your man's health. In other words if he takes ill that is time you have to spend caring for him or being without him this not only takes and emotional toll and financial toll but also a sexual one. According to The Male Health Center below is a list of common problems women share with their men when his health is failing:

ERECTILE DYSFUNCTION

The 30 million partners of men suffering from impotence suffer too, losing not only intimacy but self-esteem, many assuming that they have become unappealing or that he's cheating.

PREMATURE EJACULATION

According to recent studies, 25-30% of men ejaculate certainly within 2 to 3 minutes. This may affect many women's ability to enjoy intercourse. Additionally, studies are coming out showing tremendous negative impact on relationships, self-esteem, and even quality of life for men and their partners as a result of premature ejaculation.

SEXUALLY TRANSMITTED DISEASES

If he has a sexually transmitted disease, she probably will get it too. This is a widespread problem; one in four American adults has an incurable STD. Many STDs are more hazardous to women than men, yet are less easily detected because they occur inside the vagina. While the man's symptoms may be obvious, the women can be infected for several months before she or her doctor discovers the disease. By that time the infection may have caused pelvic inflammatory disease, a serious condition that can lead to ectopic pregnancy, infertility, or persistent pelvic pain. Also, condyloma and possibly herpes have been associated with cervical cancer, and of course, AIDS is deadly.

BIRTH CONTROL

As many women as men choose sterilization for birth control, although vasectomy is safer, less expensive and more easily reversed than tubal ligation. The reasons are male myths and ungrounded fears about vasectomy.

INFERTILITY

Male infertility may make pregnancy impossible or difficult. About 40 percent of the time, a couple's inability to conceive results from a problem in the male partner.

RISKY HEALTH HABITS

A man's risky health habits endanger his partner; smoking leads to secondhand smoking, alcoholism can lead to car accidents or abusive behavior, and so on.

DISABILITY

If he becomes disabled, chances are great she will become his primary care giver. His disability can limit a couple's social activities. Many women look forward to golfing, traveling, or visiting grandchildren with their partners during their retirement. They are concerned about their quality of life in the future.

DEATH

The ultimate effect is living alone. Because many men smoke more, drink more, don't eat a nutritious diet, visit the doctor less frequently, and generally refuse to take care of themselves, they die. As a result a woman can expect to live 7 years longer than her partner — 10 percent of the total life-span. The difference in life expectancy between a black man and a white woman is even greater, 14 years.

COACH KENYA'S RECOMMENDATIONS ON KEEPING YOUR PARTNER HEALTHY

Ladies, I know you're busy but look at keeping your man healthy as an investment in the family besides being sick involves much more down time than maintaining good health. Here are some recommendations on keeping your partner living healthier and longer:

- Be partners in the process.
- Watch for signs and symptoms.
- Let him know that you care and share information.
- Schedule regular checkups and go with him to appointments.
- Get Educated about men's health and his personal health history.
- Understand how your partner approaches the subject of health.
- Most importantly, start a routine of healthy eating and exercise today.

I realize this might seem a bit overwhelming especially if you're already dealing with chronic illness. If you are presently fighting an illness I strongly suggest you follow all the steps above along with your doctor's recommendation, in doing so, you will have a much better chance of seeing your health turn around. However I would like to urge you to start the investment of healthy eating and exercise today. Do not wait to become among the chronically ill.

Know this - your body, at your very next meal, will begin working for you to correct any damage you have done so don't wait start today.

*The best thing you can do
for poor people is
not be one of them.* [10]

-Steve Harvey's Dad

CHAPTER 6

Financial Fitness

The benefits of giving your time, talent and money is immeasurable, but the thing I like most about giving is that it means you have it to give. I can hardly wait for the time that I can consistently tithe one thousand dollars a week. For some that seems like a concept that is farfetched but looking at it from a broader perspective it is simply ten percent of ten thousand dollars. There is still nine thousand dollars left over each week so one thousand is really chump change. The Bible is filled with many verses on giving. One of my personal favorites is Deuteronomy 15:10 "you shall surely give to him, and your heart shall not be grieved when you give to him: because for this thing the lord God shall bless you in all your works and in all that you put your hand to." Let's be honest; the average person is not looking at making ten thousand dollars each week much less giving one thousand a week to a church or charity. So for the sake of argument let's look at smaller numbers. Say you bring home five hundred dollars each week then your financial contribution would be ten percent which is fifty dollars each week. Now that I have broken the math down into smaller bites I hope that it seems more doable.

What's Food Got To Do With It?

If this seems like too much or farfetched consider what your attitude is about giving. Perhaps you have gone through life never being introduced to the ideal of giving or perhaps you are always in financial defense mode because your personal finances are not where you would want them to be. If this is you this information if used correctly will change your entire life and includes your finances.

The amazing thing about givers is that they continue to receive so that five hundred dollars or any amount will likely increase if you are willing to put into to place concepts that create abundance.

Upon my return to Chicago, I immediately noticed a disconnect in social and financial karma among certain groups while others thrived even with limited resources. Were people broke because they were not valuing one another or where they not valuing one another because they where broke?

I have witnessed two types of we'll call them contributors. Understand that what you do or fail to do is still your contribution. In other words, if you're contributing nothing to a situation then your contribution is nothing. The first type of contributor either lived in a home that their parents had paid for and passed on to them or benefited in some way with subsidized housing and other government programs. At first glance one would think this was an ideal situation. A paid for home or discounted rent! Typically, a person's rent or mortgage is their largest expense. So not having this expense should allow for some major wiggle room. Even if you're a person who does not make a lot of money this set up if done correctly would allow opportunities to increase your income. Perhaps a second job or continued education would be a means of doing so or at the very least having people in the home that could contribute would provide some level of financial stability to everyone involved. On the contrary what I witnessed was there was usually one person pulling the weight for everyone. And because the other players in the equation were not held to a higher standard no one in the household benefitted. In essence a situation like this if handled correctly could provide an express route out of poverty. However, more often than not, these arrangements lack structure and commitment leaving the main contributor feeling stuck in a deep hole.

The other type of contributor is twofold. This type of giver usually accomplished an above the status quo level of financial success usually due to higher education, military experience or just plain old hard work. They give of their time and talents but found themselves surrounded by so many non-givers that their efforts appear mute. Or they reached a level of success usually with very little support from their immediate circle that lead to burn out. Thus choosing to separate themselves from their community taking their time, talent and finances abroad.

Now let's be clear I do not judge in fact I can see clearly how good people could fall into either of these scenarios. I encourage you to take inventory of what type of contributor you are realizing that there is always room for improvement. Being a giver is not about giving the biggest prize or where you are at the moment it is all about where you are trusting God to go.

We need one another's time, talents and yes finances to grow and thrive. Be a giver!

COACH KENYA'S RECOMMENDATION ON CREATING FINANCIAL FITNESS

I have certainly had my share of financial ups and downs. I'll be first to admit that the ups are a heck of a lot more pleasant than the downs. Over the years I have listened to a few financial experts. One in particular has provided me with sound advice that is doable. I highly recommend Dave Ramsey for financial advice he offers a host of products and services to help you climb out of a financial rut. Everything from starting an emergency fund to learning how to be a giver is included in his comprehensive programs. If you are serious about your financial future take a few minutes to look at what it would take to start building a sound financial future now. Go to WWW.DAVERAMSEY.COM for a complete list of financial products, services and broadcast.

As a Health Coach I remind my clients just as you would give your body time to turn itself around and replace bad habits for healthy habits, financial health is the same. First understand exactly where you are and where you want to go and then get the correct information on how to get there. It won't happen overnight but if you faithfully continue, it will happen. Remember certain things equal certain things.

The causes of obesity are varied and complex, but the lack of daily physical activity is an important factor. [11]

—Risa Lavizzo-Mourey

CHAPTER 7

Exercise Is A Bonus

What the hell are ya'll doing? A study from our friends at the Centers for Disease Control (CDC) shows that eighty percent of American adults are not getting the recommended amount of weekly exercise. This means you are setting yourself up for chronic illness. Now let's be clear exercise is a bonus. If you had to pick between eating right and exercise well I think by now you know which one I would opt for. The truth is you do not have to pick you can have them both. A diet full of nutritious foods and physical fitness that includes cardio and strength training are well within reach.

It is recommended that children get at least one hour per day of psychical exercise and adults two hours and thirty minutes each week. I am not going to let the adults off the hook quite that easy. The truth is if the adults are not getting their fair share of exercise their children are likely lacking too. Here is the deal anyone who practices self-love and self-care can get in 30 minutes of exercise five days per week. Over time I like to see that thirty minutes increase to forty, fifty and even sixty minutes five days each week. I mean really you are already engaged in the activity you may as well get the most out of it.

BENEFITS OF EXERCISE

Let me offer you a different perspective on exercise. Let's say you completed a special project at work and now it's bonus time. The boss comes to give you your bonus check and you refuse it. You simply do not want it. Sounds silly right? If you are working on practicing self-love and eating right, exercise is the bonus that ties it all together. Exercise has many health benefits from anti-aging to better sex. With so many forms of exercise available anyone can find an activity that they enjoy and don't mind sticking to. Here is a list of the common benefits of exercise:

- Heart health
- Helps with mood
- Helps regulate sleep
- Helps control weight
- Personal time out for yourself
- Promotes better sleep
- Provides a healthy outlet for stress
- Promotes great looking skin, hair and nails

The most common excuse is I don't have time for exercise. The most common response is will you have time for hospital visits? Another common excuse is I don't have money for a membership. In my health coaching practice weight loss clients spend a large majority of time working out using their own body weight. When the weather is nice we take our workouts outdoors and add a brisk walk to the routine. You don't have to spend money for membership dues. Here as a list of body weight exercises from BODY DIVINE™ that you can do anywhere without purchasing a gym membership:

COACH KENYA'S FAVORITE BODY WEIGHT EXERCISES

Cardio or Warm Up	Time	Sets/Reps
Running in place	1 minute	Warm up or in between rounds
Jumping rope	1 minute	Warm up or in between rounds
Jumping jacks	1 minute	Warm up or in between rounds
Up down pushups	1 minute	Warm up or in between rounds
Side knee side	1 minute	Warm up or in between rounds
Side to side shuffles	1 minute	Warm up or in between rounds
Front/side/back kicks	1 minute	Warm up or in between rounds

CORE	Time	Sets/Reps
Babies aka Russian Twist	1 minute	3 sets
Bicycles	1 minute	3 sets
Leg Ups	1 minute	3 sets
Plank Hold	1 minute	3 sets

LEGS	Time	Sets/Reps
Burpees	NA	3 sets/15 reps
Frog Squats	NA	3 sets/15 reps
Walking Lunges	NA	3 sets/15 reps
Runners shuffle	NA	3 sets/15 reps

ARMS & UPPER	Time	Sets/Reps
Punch side twist	NA	3 sets/15 reps
Upper cuts	NA	3 sets/15 reps
Push ups (varied)	NA	3 sets/15 reps
Dips	NA	3 sets/15 reps

Pick one exercise from each category and see how you do. Go at your own pace but challenge yourself if it is too easy add an extra exercise or increase speed and intensity. Work out for a minimum of thirty minutes then gradually increase your time to forty and then sixty minutes. Anything over sixty minutes is overkill. Remember exercise is a bonus and proper nutrition through primary and secondary foods is ninety percent of living a healthy lifestyle.

Nothing happens until something moves.[12]

-Einstein

CHAPTER 8

Exactly What to Do Now!

So what now? You have read the information and nine times out of ten you have heard it all before. Your awareness has been raised. The next few pages are filled with step-by-step instructions to assist you in starting where you are without fear of failure. Now it is time to start your own personal wellness practice. Remember to do what works best for you. Not everyone is the same. First, let's get things in the proper perspective. As a coach I know it's hard to get people to eat their peas and carrots and do pushup when their lives are chaotic. Let's look at other wellness components you'll want to practice to tie things together and create balance in every part of your life.

FAITH

Spiritual Energy

Gratitude

RELATIONSHIPS

Family, Friends & Food

Career

Intimacy

MOVEMENT

Passions

Relaxation

Physical Activity

Invest in your Community

FINANCIAL FITNESS

Be a Giver

Financial Literacy

Discipline

Next follow these three steps:

Step 1 – SHOP

Make a list and go shopping. Do not overdo it! Grab a week's worth of groceries and remember to focus on vegetables and some fruits as your primary source of nutrients. Add in proteins, grains and fats in smaller amounts. Weigh yourself before you start. Decide on a timeline (I recommend a minimum of 30 days) and don't worry about being perfect just progressive. You will be astonished by the mental and physical transformation you will experience in a short period of time.

Step 2 – PREP

Prepare an assortment of raw and cooked produce. Prepare enough for three to four days and throw them in zip lock bags or storage containers. Do not over complicate things; remember God already did the work. Your job is to have fun with different combinations of food. The key is to have them handy.

Step 3 – EAT

Get in three square meals each day! And yes, it is important to eat breakfast and break the fast. This does not mean you have to step out of bed and eat but by all means make every attempt to eat something at least an hour after waking.

Now that you have wholesome foods on hand and a mindset to eat a minimum of breakfast, lunch and dinner, the next step is to look at your plate. Do not over think the process just follow a few simple rules when plating your food. The next page contains what a BODY DIVINE™ plate should consist of. Remember we do not put restrictions on food; we simply manage how we eat them. Knowing that everything we put in our body either helps or hurts.

What's Food Got To Do With It?

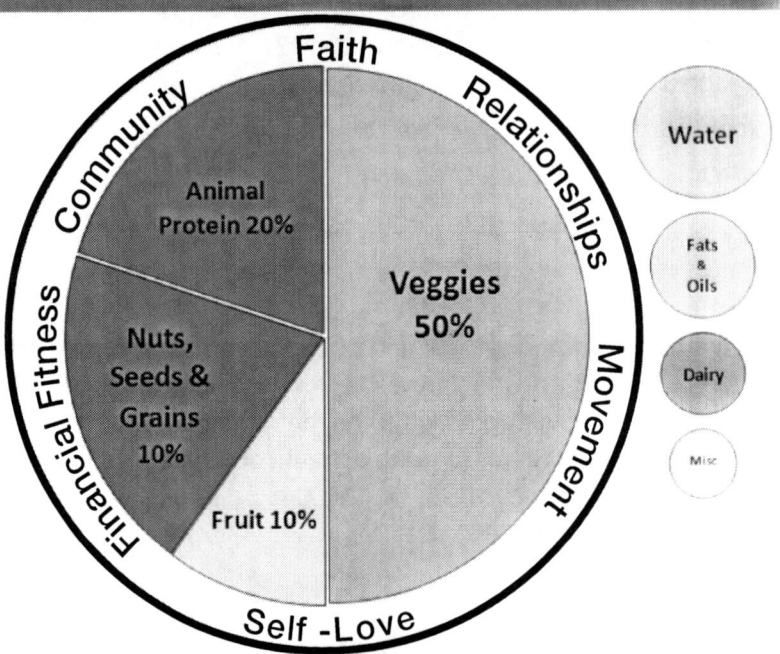

Coach Kenya Catlin

10 Easy Grab & Go Snacks
from the Body Divine Cookbook

Nut and Berry Medley	Cucumber Lime Salad
2 tbs. Almond butter 6 Strawberries ½ Cup blueberries	½ Cucumber 6 Cherry tomatoes ½ Avocado Trace of EVOO, lime, sea salt
Chocolaty Nut Delight	**Kale and Pineapple Salad**
4 Dark chocolate cashews 1 Bartlett pear 1 oz. Walnuts	1 cup Kale (chopped) 2 oz. Pineapple Trace of EVOO, lemon, sea salt
Summer Spinach Salad	**Steamed Cabbage with Apples**
1 cup Spinach (raw) 6 Strawberries 1 oz. Walnuts Trace of EVOO, lime, sea salt	1 cup Cabbage, sautéed in EVOO Topped with sliced apple and walnut
Celery and Hummus Sticks	**Broccoli Medley Bags**
2 large pc. Celery ½ Zucchini 4 Asparagus spears 2 oz. Hummus for dipping	6 Broccoli flowerets 6 Cauliflower flowerets 10 Grapes
Sunny Seed Breakfast	**BODY DIVINE™ Trail Mix**
½ Grapefruit 2 oz. Sunflower seeds 1 small Banana	1 oz. almonds, walnuts, pumpkin seeds ½ oz. dark or milk chocolate squares ½ oz. Sesame sticks ½ oz. Cranberries

God already did the work. Keep snack foods handy and eat variety of proteins, carbs and fat.

Healthy Low-Carb Snacks

Avocado Turkey with Green Onion & Mini peppers	Spinach & Artichoke Dip with **Chicken Breast**
Chicken Liver Pate and Raw Veggies with Ranch Dressing	Celery Sticks and Almond Butter
Sardines Cheese and Grape Tomatoes	Roast Beef Asparagus Horseradish Sauce
Cream Cheese Stuffed Mini Peppers Wrapped with Scallops & Bacon	Broccoli and Cauliflower With Bean Dip
Hummus Raw Veggie Mix Salmon	Tuna with mayo Pita and Zucchini Chips Pickle

Go for it! There are no rules try different combinations of real foods.

Healthy Drink Ideas

Banana Nut Smoothie 6oz Almond Milk 1 small Banana 1 to 2oz Mixed Nuts 1 tbsp Coconut Oil or EVOO Top with a Shake of Cinnamon	Green Tea Kool Aide 12oz Green Tea A shake of Crystal Light (any flavor) Fresh Mint Lemon or Lime Wedge Serve on Ice
Ginger Water 12 oz Green Tea or Water 1oz Fresh Ginger 1oz Mint Cucumber Slices *Let fresh ingredients marinate in liquid and enjoy.*	Veggie Smoothie 6oz Green Tea 1 cup Kale or Spinach ½ Cucumber 2 oz. Pineapple 4 medium strawberries 1 tbsp Coconut Oil or EVOO

A Really Green Veggie Smoothie
6 oz Green Tea or Water
1 cup Kale or Spinach
½ Cucumber
1 piece celery
2oz tomato
2oz carrots
1oz parsley
1 small Apple
1oz Ginger
1 tbsp Coconut Oil or EVOO
Top with a drizzle of honey and a Shake of Cinnamon

Remember that liquids are not intended to replace meals.

For more information about BODY DIVINE™ weight loss, recipes, culinary classes or healthy eating workshops go to

WWW.MYBODYDIVINE.COM
or Contact Coach KENYA at
INFO@MYBODYDIVINE.COM

GET MOVING!

Cardio or Warm Up	Time	Sets/Reps
Running in place	1 minute	Warm up or in between rounds
Jumping rope	1 minute	Warm up or in between rounds
Jumping jacks	1 minute	Warm up or in between rounds
Up down pushups	1 minute	Warm up or in between rounds
Side knee side	1 minute	Warm up or in between rounds
Side to side shuffles	1 minute	Warm up or in between rounds
Front/side/back kicks	1 minute	Warm up or in between rounds

CORE	Time	Sets/Reps
Babies aka Russian Twist	1 minute	3 sets
Bicycles	1 minute	3 sets
Leg Ups	1 minute	3 sets
Plank Hold	1 minute	3 sets

LEGS	Time	Sets/Reps
Burpees	NA	3 sets/15 reps
Frog Squats	NA	3 sets/15 reps
Walking Lunges	NA	3 sets/15 reps
Runners shuffle	NA	3 sets/15 reps

ARMS & UPPER	Time	Sets/Reps
Punch side twist	NA	3 sets/15 reps
Upper cuts	NA	3 sets/15 reps
Push ups (varied)	NA	3 sets/15 reps
Dips	NA	3 sets/15 reps

Pick a exercise from each category and follow the recommended reps and sets. Try to work up to 30 minutes at least three days each week.

*I ~~hope~~,
nope pray
this helps.
    —Coach Kenya*

Footnotes & Quotes

1. Lucado, Max. *The Devotional Bible*. 2003.

2. Donne, John. "No Man Is an Island". www.poemhunter.com. 2015.

3. Percentage of adults ages 18 to 64 with any chronic condition or disability. The Commonwealth Fund. 2015.

4. Percentage of adults 18 to 64 who are overweight or obese. The Commonwealth Fund. 2015.

5. "What's in a Cigarette?". American Lung Association. www.lung.org. 2015.

6. *Healthier sources of caffeine.* WebMD. www.webmd.com. 2015.

7. Keys, Alicia. "Element of Freedom". www.metrolyrics.com. 2009.

8. Alauda, Astrid. "The 50 Best Quotes About Health & Nutrition". www.globalhealingcenter.com . 2011.

9. Brillat-Savarin, Jean Anthelme. http://www.brainyquote.com. 2015.

10. Steve Harvey's Dad. Tampa Bay Times. www.thetampabay.com. 2011.

11. Lavizzo-Mourey, Risa. Brainy Quote. www.brainyquote.com. 2015.

12. Einstein, Albert. Good Reads. www.goodreads.com. 2015.

References

Lucado, Max. *The Devotional Bible*. 2003. Print

Whitney Houston. *The Greatest Love of All*. 1985. CD

Walter Hawkins and Family. *Be Grateful*. 1978. CD

"What Is Chronic Disease?" *The Center for Managing Chronic Disease*. The University of Michigan, 2011. Web. 2015

"Diet and Nutrition Prevention of Chronic Diseases." *Green Facts*. Green Facts. Web. 2015

"Red Wine and Resveratrol: Good for Your Heart?" *Heart Disease*. Mayo Foundation for Medical Education and Research, 2015. Web. 2015

"A Brief History of Tobacco." *CNN*. Cable News Network, 2000. Web. 2015

"What's in a Cigarette?" *American Lung Association*. American Lung Association, 2015. Web. 2015

"History of Caffeine." The Caffeine Page. The Caffeine Page, 2015. Web. 2015

"Macronutrients: The Importance of Carbohydrate, Protein, and Fat." *McKinley Health Center*. The Board of Trustees of the University of Illinois, 2014. Web. 2015

Lehman, Shereen. "Micronutrients." *About Health*. About.com, 2015. Web. 2015

"Physical Differences Between Men and Women." *Dr. James Dobson's Family Talk*. Dr. James Dobson's Family Talk, 2015. Web. 2015

"How Women Can Help Men Stay Healthy." *The Male Health Center*. The Male Health Center, 2006. Web. 2015

ABOUT THE AUTHOR

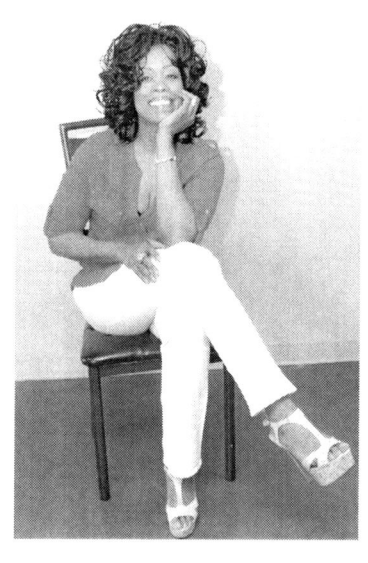

Coach KENYA Catlin is a Certified Health & Wellness Coach Practitioner, Motivational Speaker and Author who assists individuals, communities, corporations and municipalities in pursuing healthier lives in an effort to prevent & manage chronic illness by teaching the practical principals of proper nutrition, fitness and overall wellness through behavior modifications. Coach KENYA started her practice in 2007 and has achieved long-term sustainable results.

About the BODY DIVINE™

Since 2007, BODY DIVINE™ has been assisting everyday people in becoming better by utilizing "A Comprehensive Approach" to Wellness through proper nutrition, fitness, weight loss and a host of other wellness products. Our programs provide people with all the tools they need to live a healthier happier life.

My Mission is to revolutionize the healthcare industry by offering comprehensive programs and services that are attainable to all.

My Vision is to accomplish the mission by having fun, building community and putting people to work in the ever growing field of preventative healthcare.

Become a Health Coach

In addition, Health Coaching is here to stay offering a myriad of opportunities. If you think assisting individuals, groups, churches, municipalities and businesses in creating long-term sustainable wellness is for you, I welcome you to explore becoming a Health Coach.

For more information about BODY DIVINE™ products and services or to become a Health Coach go to WWW.MYBODYDIVINE.COM or Contact Coach KENYA at Kenyacatlin@gmail.com

CPSIA information can be obtained at www.ICGtesting.com
Printed in the USA
LVOW11s0603170715

446377LV00001B/2/P